Dr. Kelly Smith

My Pants Don't Hurt Anymore

ISBN: 1-4392-6514-3

ISBN-13: 9781439265147

Table of Contents

Introduction

Let me introduce myself. My name is Doctor Kelly Smith. I am a full time physician, and a part time college professor. I am also less than a year away from 50 and about the same number of pounds overweight.

This book was never intended to be a book at all. If someone told me it would be published I would have thought them to be simple-minded. I had an idea on how to lose weight quickly and although I was not looking to set the world on fire, or write a book, I did want to test some theories and lose weight, quick and painlessly.

At first in my quest to lose weight, if I had any questions I just asked my colleagues. Unfortunately, their answers were the same rhetoric that I had been hearing all of my life. It quickly dawned on me that people cling to what they have heard in the past.

The only real ground breaking work in the world of Diet and Nutrition was when Dr. Robert Atkins set the world on its ear with his revolutionary views and ideas about nutrition and weight loss. The inescapable fact was that if I really wanted to know the answers to theories and questions that I had, I would have to find them out for myself. That is how this book came about.

I designed a weight loss plan that was to last a total of two weeks, and kept a daily journal of what I learned, and experienced along the way. Most importantly I kept track of how much weight I lost and how quickly I lost it. The end result was that I came up with a plan that defied conventional weight loss by combining fasting and dieting. I have cleverly called this plan the Fast Diet.

Another glaring difference with my book vs. others is that it is not loaded with a lot of verbiage to make it appear like a tome of the ancient pharaohs. In reading other dieting and fasting books, without fail after about thirty pages into the book I, like many others, skip to the back to find the diet plan. It is not that their data or information is not correct, it is just irrelevant. I didn't like biochemistry or organic chemistry when I had to take it in school while working on my doctor ate. I certainly don't want to force others to do the same while reading my book.

I did ask the opinion of others and they said that I should make the book as technical as possible to lend it credibility, and give it weight. I didn't really want to, but once again I began to fall into the trap of doing what is expected as opposed to what I thought I should do. Fortunately I let my mom and dad read the rough draft and told them that I still had a lot of "filler", to add to make the book seem more important. My dad asked me why I wanted to do that, and I told him what everyone else had told me, *to make people take it seriously*. My dad then told me that if he was looking at a "How To", book that was super thick, he would be intimidated and wouldn't attempt it.

After hearing those words, I went back through the book and took out the "filler." The last thing that I wanted was for someone to have any more reasons not to lose weight. This journey was to make losing weight quick and easy, not to explain the atomic structure of a watermelon.

When I began my Fast Diet, I purposely stacked the deck against myself. I am slightly obsessive. I tend to count things, like wheels on semi-trucks. I know it makes no sense, but it keeps me occupied when I drive. One of the other things I do is read the fine print on things like medicine and weight loss products. I constantly see these screaming headlines, *I lost 50 pounds by using Fat Away,* or *take one of these supplements and lose a pound a day* or my favorite, *lose 20 pounds without trying.*

My challenge to you is next time you see one of these ads on TV or in a magazine, read the fine print. This is what you will see, "results *not* typical and may vary with the individual". The other hidden message goes something like this; *Suzy Sunshine lost 40 pounds by taking Fat Away with exercise and diet.* Now I am not the sharpest tool in the shed, but I am pretty positive I could achieve those same results by taking supplements filled with sand as long as I dieted and exercised. If I liked or was even willing to engage in exercise and diet, I would not be in the shape I am in now. I would not be writing this book on how to lose weight, because I would not need to. I would certainly not be filled with biblical fire because I took some pill to race out and join the gym.

Most people are motivated on the first day of any activity when they don't need any encouragement. I have joined the gym lots of times. The first week I am motivated and excited to be getting back into shape again. It is not till the next few weeks were I begin to taper off and eventually quit. The same holds true with a diet. I have a bad habit of talking myself out of things that I don't really want to do, even if I know it is good for me.

If I run, it doesn't matter if it is one mile or three miles. Until I hit the half way point of the run I struggle. The thought that runs through my head is that every step I take is one step farther that I have to take to get back home. After the half way point I am fine. It is just the opposite mantra running through my head. Every step I take is one step closer to finishing.

For a diet plan to be successful for me, I had to come up with a means of getting around the first half of the diet. If I didn't do this I would be stuck in the same cycle of wanting to quit before I achieved my goal. Take it from me coming up with a plan that didn't have a beginning was *tough*. It sounds like an oxymoron and a paradox all rolled together, but that is what I did. That is why the Fast Diet only begins with three days of melon fasting before you can eat.

Something motivated you to not only want to lose weight, but do something about it. Unfortunately just like the gym, the first day or two of the diet is no problem. It is the next few days when you find yourself cheating and eventually quitting. It is my hope that as you read this book you will put aside all of your pre-conceived notions of what to expect with a diet. Truly this is not a diet in the classic sense of the word. There are days when you can eat whatever you want, including beer and dark chocolate. Let your conscious be your guide.

As I stated earlier, this originally began as a tracking journal, so it may seem slightly disjointed at first. But one of the wonderful things about this format is that the day I experienced something unexpected, I would write about it that day.

This allows you to use the book not only as a guide, but also as a timeline to prepare you as you encounter some of the problems I did. Above all learn from my mistakes. As you read this you will see the mistakes I made were more than a few. The food that I find appropriate for this plan is all melons. So, let's get started...

Chapter One

The Journal – A Test for the Plan: Charting the Successes and Failures

The goal of this chapter is to share with you the steps and missteps that I encountered as I began this journey. I hope that by reading about my experiences, I can save you the problems that occurred as I tested my theory.

Tuesday, February 17

I start my weight loss plan tomorrow. So of course I went to a steak restaurant and had a giant T-bone with all of the fixin's, as a last Hoorah.

Today is February 17th; my weight today at the start is 233 lbs. I am going to follow a weight loss plan that I have devised for the next two weeks. I have no goal of how much weight I am going to lose because I have no idea how much it will be. My only parameters are that I am going to stick with it for two weeks. At the end of that time I will see what has happened.

The First Three Days
Wednesday, February 18

I started my Fast Diet on Wednesday the 18th of February.

Wednesday morning I had a half glass of 2 percent milk, and stopped at a fast food restaurant and ordered a large unsweetened tea. I think it was a 32 oz cup. I sipped on the tea for the rest of the day. I took my blood pressure and it was fine, 122/78.

I took it around four o'clock in the afternoon. At around 7:00 p.m. I had a half of a small seedless watermelon. I then had my daughter take a picture of me without my shirt on. It was humiliating. At about 9:30 p.m. I had a cup of hot tea with milk and honey.

Thursday, February 19

I skipped the milk for breakfast and took some vitamins and fiber supplements with a mouthful of water. Stopped for my unsweetened tea and went to the office. I weighed myself and was stunned to see that I now weighed 229 lbs. I don't really believe that it is all water weight since I had massive amounts of water intake from the watermelon. Even if it was just water weight, so what. I was lighter and my pants fit better. I then went home for lunch at 12:30 p.m. and had half of a honeydew melon. I had supper at 7:30 p.m. which consisted of 1/4 of the left over honeydew and half of a cantaloupe. At around 9:00 p.m. I had a tea with milk and honey, I had another tea around 11:30 p.m..

Friday, February 20

I am still not hungry. I am really surprised by that. I had a couple of mouthfuls of honeydew and my vitamins with a cup of water. Once again I bought my large unsweetened tea to sip on throughout the day. I got to work and approached the scale. I was actually very anxious as well as excited. I did not know if day one was a fluke or if I would continue to lose weight or regress and gain weight. I had already convinced myself that my clothes were heavier today than yesterday just in case I gained.

I stepped on the scale and my weight is now 227. My lunch and supper were a repeat of yesterday. The melons were not very ripe so I am just trying to finish them up for lunch. I had a 1/4 of cantaloupe and an 1/8 of the honeydew. I also had two 3oz liquid yogurts. Supper was one half of a medium sized watermelon. I had planned on going to the Chinese buffet Saturday to satisfy my cravings. Fortunately I don't really have any cravings. So we will see.

I have been giving the question of why I don't have any cravings a lot of thought. I think I have finally come up with a working hypothesis and theory. It is my contention that I am not having any cravings, because I am not eating "linkage food," by this I mean foods that are associated with other foods, i.e. meat and potatoes, ham and cheese sandwiches, pancakes and syrup. That is why with most diets even though we are physically full, we have the craving for something else like gravy over your meat.

❧ ❧ ❧

A NOTE TO MY READERS:

Our brain automatically links certain foods together and when we don't get them we miss them. The melons that I am eating they are a "stand-alone" food. When we want watermelon, we just want watermelon. So when we eat a bowl or 1/4 of a melon and become full, there is no signal from our brain saying ok, time for the rest of our meal. Our stomach is allowed to tell our brain we are full now, and our brain can look at our stomach and its established linkages and say "yep that's right".

This allows us to walk away from the kitchen without the feeling of something left undone. Another great thing about using the melons for this plan is that melons are traditionally dessert. In this way we condition our brain to our benefit. Everybody knows that you don't get to eat your desert until you are through with your meal. Like Pink Floyd said "You don't get your pudding if you don't eat your meat". Now the brain is tricked into thinking that it has just had a seven course meal.

The brain takes inventory of the body and runs through its check list:

	Yes	NO
Did we eat?	_____ *	_____
Are we Hungry?	_____	_____ *
Are we full?	_____ *	_____
Did we have desert?	_____ *	_____
Are we done?	_____ *	_____

When all of the proper columns have been checked in the appropriate space the brain is able to move onto something else. There is no more feeling like you have been cheated out of something.

And On the Fourth Day...
Saturday, February 21

I started to get hit with my cravings last night. They began about 8:00 p.m. and lasted till 11:00 p.m.. After that I was fine. I think the reason for my cravings was that I have planned from day one to binge on Saturday. I believe that knowing that I will eat on Saturday was making me hungry about the things that I want.

I went to the office today and weighed myself. I lost another two lbs. I am now down to 225. I am very pleased. That is 8 pounds. in three days. I still plan on eating today, because it was on my schedule to do so. I also have a theory that if I surprise my system with food after so long it will shock it into overdrive on digestion and processing of the stored fat.

Today got a little out of hand. I had to go to my kids martial arts meet today and didn't get to eat anything till 3:30 p.m.

I had a slice of pizza and a root beer with a candy bar. Later, at about 5:30 p.m. I made a giant bowl of tuna salad about the size of two cereal bowls, and grazed on it for hours. About 10:00 p.m. my throat was kind of sore from cheering my kids at the tournament so I had an ice cream sandwich and a cup of hot tea and honey. And just because I could, I had another soda to soothe my sore throat. That justified me buying the ice cream and drinking the soda. One surprising phenomenon was that I actually wanted some more melon. I thought I would be sick of the sight of it, but I am pleasantly surprised that I am actually kind of craving it. I refused to eat it though. Monday will be here soon enough, so I am enjoying the comfort foods while I can.

I expect to gain weight tomorrow; I just have to see what it is. Sunday is also scheduled as an eat day. However it is to be a responsible day of eating, No ice cream and doughnuts, or Soda.

Sunday February 22nd,

Saturday was kind of a weird night. As I was lying in bed my stomach was rumbling and grumbling like there was no tomorrow. I didn't realize that for the last couple of days I had not been having any stomach noises. That struck me as kind of odd until I realized that my body was busy breaking down stored fat instead of spending all of its energy on digestion.

I weighed today. The damage wasn't as bad as I had thought. I did gain weight but only 3/4 pound. My weight is now back up to 225 3/4 lbs.

I am still going to eat responsibly today, but will probably get popcorn when I go to the movie. After all I am only human.

Monday February 23rd,

It was a horrible idea to start eating again. Once my feeding button was pushed I didn't stop, just knowing that Monday I would not be able to eat again made me eat everything that I could find. It was like ordering shots when the bartender tells you it is last call. I ate everything - popcorn, a ham, egg, and cheese croissant, lemon-filled doughnut, more tuna fish, chili, a couple of candy bars, and on and on.

Normally I have to think really hard as to why I respond in certain ways, but not this time. This was the classic psychological phenomenon of "the fear of loss," Knowing that I would curtail my ability to eat on Monday set off a psychological need to hoard. Even though I knew that I was only giving up things for a couple of days was not enough to stop the cycle. Did I say cycle? It was more like trying to shut off a water fall. You would think that this was bad enough, but it wasn't. My response was compounded. After going for three days without eating and then eating all of that tuna fish, the next day my digestive tract was in an uproar. My stomach hurt, I had gas and diarrhea. I had expected to have diarrhea during the fast portion while eating all of those melons, but it never happened. Anyway I am a big subscriber of comfort foods, and since I felt bad, I ate junk to make me feel better. Of course that didn't work either. It was like trying to drown a fish with water.

In a way it was a good thing that this happened. One, it showed that I am not superman, and two, it pointed out to me that losing weight not only has physiological factors to overcome such as "linkage food," but I have to be aware of the routine habits such as, *I need coffee so I won't be cranky, therefore if I drink coffee I am a happier person.* Of course there is no basis for this. If I choose to be cranky or happy it is up to me, it has nothing to do with the beverage. I believe it therefore it must be true. Perception is reality, there are a million sayings and all of them are true.

Now to the bad news. I am back to 229. I still think that after eating again my body will jump start the process of digestion and burning off stored fat again. But it is still depressing getting on the scale and seeing that my weight had gone up again. That stupid little machine so influences my mood it is ridiculous. I have been happy all week. I have been walking around with my shirt off, thinking I look pretty good. I even flexed a few times in front of the mirror. This is all something I haven't done in ages. As a matter of fact I have become something of a Vampire. Even though I use a mirror to brush my teeth and shave, I realized that I had quit seeing myself. I am sure that this is some kind of defense because who wants to see the fat guy? In my mind I still look like I did in my thirties. I have no reason for reality to rear its ugly head and ruin my good mood.

Even though I have had a few surprises, So far I have been mostly correct in my assumptions and hypotheses. I am looking forward to Tuesday so I can weigh myself again.

I had planned on letting Tuesday be a cheat day. Tuesday is my day off and the wife and I usually go to the movies while the kids are in school. I personally think it is sacrilegious to sit in a movie without popcorn and a soda. But after this weekend, I think that I am going to skip the cheat day and either not go to the movies or go but just not buy anything.

Tuesday, February 24th,

Well it wasn't as good as I had hoped. I lost a pound yesterday and am now back to 227. I had been expecting a much bigger decline. I had a half of a medium sized watermelon, and one half of a cantaloupe yesterday as well as vitamins and two 3-ounce yogurts for the health of my immune and digestive system. I have stopped listing fiber supplements as one of the things that I take in the morning. The reason is simple, I don't need them. I thought with all of the fluid I was taking in that I would have diarrhea. That has not happened so I see no need for the extra fiber. Even though I stuck to my guns yesterday and didn't nibble on anything it was very hard. The wife decided to cook lasagna for the kids. All of a sudden that half of watermelon didn't seem nearly as desirable as it was a minute ago.

I had to physically leave the kitchen. I went up and soaked in the tub until all of the plates were cleared from the table. Again I want to reiterate. I am nothing special. I have no special willpower abilities. If I did I would not have been fat through my forties. I say this not as an excuse but to give anyone reading this hope. I mentioned earlier that I was planning on having this as a cheat day.

But after only losing a pound, I am going to skip it and continue on the Fast. Since I have basically started this fast twice, once when I began and again yesterday after my gluttony period, I have learned that the hardest day is Day One.

Having lived through a couple of mistakes, I am going to only allow *one* day of gluttony. After reviewing my notes the weight gain after one day was insignificant. It is combining two days worth of binging that caused all of my problems and set me back about 3 or 4 pounds.

People have asked me why I even have one day of gluttony in my program. The answer is simple, when I originally started the Fast Diet, I thought eating in the middle would jump start the digestive system and burn stored reserves that much quicker. That was true, but deep down I know that the other reason that I added those days was that I didn't think I could go for the full two weeks, without breaking down and having a couple of meals. Even now, after having stopped the fast for two days with miserable results, I am not willing to completely cut out a food day. Again this is not geared toward the athletes and body builders who think nothing of getting out of bed at five o'clock in the morning to go running before work. I simply don't have that kind of commitment. Knowing that in a couple of days I will be able to eat makes staying on the Fast much easier for me.

I also believe that this is why diets don't work for most people in general and me in particular. The end of the tunnel on a traditional diet is too far away and much too dark at the end for me to have any hope of completing it.

I expect to lose about 20 pounds by the end of my two week Fast. Whether I don't and come up short, or I exceed the 20 pound mark, I know that I am quitting two weeks from the day I started. That is a definite time frame. There are no 'maybes' or 'I hopes' in the plan. It is simple; you fast on melons for fourteen days. At the end of that time you are done. Of course if you want to do it longer and lose more weight that is up to you.

If I was on a diet, and my goal was to lose 20 pounds, I would have no idea when that time would come. For all I know it could take me four months to lose 20 pounds by the conventional means. Now I am faced with disappointment every day. Every day I step on the scale whether I am losing weight or not I see how much farther I have to go to reach my goal. It doesn't matter if I am consistently losing weight. All I can see is how far I still have to go. I hate to admit this but I am easily discouraged. I begin to start thinking, *it has taken me two weeks to lose 4 pounds, so that means that I still have at least a month and a half left.* That is when thoughts like; *why bother - I have been fat this long we will try again later in the summer* start to kick in, and I rationalize myself out of the diet. Instead with the Fast Diet, I am actually looking forward to the next day to see how much I have lost, as well as knowing that I am one day closer to the end. This appears to be a much more productive form of motivation than just setting some nebulous goal of losing 20 pounds.

Wednesday, February 25,

I lost another pound yesterday. I am now down to 226. I did not use Tuesday as a cheat day. I just could not justify it. If I hadn't binged on the weekend and put all of those pounds back on I would be much closer to my goal of twenty pounds. I could kick myself. Not only did I set myself back by gaining 4 pounds but the time I spent losing it again could have been spent getting thinner and thinner. Since I am not "dieting," but am Fast/Dieting, for a specific period, that weekend will eventually cost me about 8 pounds. And I am here to tell you there is a big difference between 213 and 221 pounds.

I had a cantaloupe and one half today and three, 3oz liquid yogurts, and two hot teas with milk and honey.

Yesterday was harder than normal for me to stay on the fast. Since it was my day off, I was at home all day surrounded by food. I wasn't hungry, but the habit of grazing the kitchen was very strong. I am also depressed still from the weekend binge. This caused a whole new set of problems for me. My body and mind are used to being fed comfort food when depressed. From around 1:00p.m. until 4 :00 p.m. I found myself opening and closing the refrigerator like I am used to doing. Because it is habit for me to open the fridge and take something out, I had three of my liquid yogurts. .At least I was able to guide my hand toward something healthy and non-fattening. More importantly the yogurt is on my Fast plan so I didn't cheat.

Again I am constantly amazed at how something so simple as my weight going up vs. going down can affect my whole mental outlook. Before the "Weekend From Hell," I would lie in bed fantasizing (yes, sad but true), about the weight I was going to lose by tomorrow. After the binge, I am now depressed every time I get on the scale, because I still have not lost all of the 4 pounds yet. If everything stays on track I should be back to ground zero tomorrow. From that point on I should get excited again, since I will be charting new territory on the weight loss scale.

I guess I could look at this as a good thing since I know now, that there is no such thing as just a "little" cheating. I also don't have much desire to start eating again. But I am not that big of a person. I still think it stinks royally that I ate all of that food and put on that weight.

Thursday, February 26,

Time to weigh again. I am apprehensive about this weigh in. I didn't cheat or anything, but this is the day that I expect to be back to what I was before the binge. If I am right I should feel great, if I am wrong I am going to be moping around all day. Deep down I think I will make my mark. Last night I was full of energy and even did a couple of sets of bicep curls in front of the TV.

As I have mentioned previously, I am purposely not exercising. I don't want to skew the results, and personally I don't like any cardio exercise except for surfing. I know it is massively beneficial; I just don't like taking the time to do it. I also know that if I did it now my weight loss would be much more dramatic. The one thing that I don't want is a weight loss plan that has to include diet <u>and</u> exercise in order to work. Like I said earlier, even a cake and doughnut diet would work if you exercised enough. However, be that as it may, I had so much energy that I had to do something. This energy surplus is quite a pleasant surprise to me.

Today was a milestone for me. I am now down to 224 pounds. I lost 2 more pounds since yesterday. I have returned to the uncharted weight loss area. Yesterday I had 3/4 of a small watermelon, unsweetened tea, yogurt, two hot teas with milk and honey and vitamins and mineral supplements. I am going to just eat watermelon today and see if the watermelon is a greater accelerant for weight loss than the other kinds of melons that I am eating.

In all probability the real reason I lost 2 pounds yesterday was it just took my body three days to finally use and expel all of the food from the weekend. I doubt that it had anything to do with the type of melon that I ate. I can't see there being a huge difference between watermelon and honeydew, or some other type of melons. That weekend is going to haunt me till the end of time.

I keep looking at my weight and should be ecstatic. I have only fasted for a total of six days and have lost 9 pounds. That is a pound and a half a day. That is very good. I am also convinced that if I added exercise to the plan it would be even more weight loss per day. But unfortunately all that I can think about is if I hadn't gained those 4 pounds, I would now be down to 220. But not only did I go backwards by 4 pounds but I then had to lose it again. So instead of being 224 now I would be sitting on 216 pounds. And that would average out to over 2 pounds a day.

Now that I am at the half way point of my fast, I feel that there is something that I need to address. There seems to be some kind of folk lore, or legend out there that the first 10 pounds that you lose during a fast is just water weight. This came as something as a shock to me as I had never heard that before. Maybe because I was never on a fast or even cared that much about one, I was not exposed to the gossip. However now that I am up to my ears in one I am polling, reading and just plain listening to people talk about their pre-conceived concepts. Quite honestly I am stunned.

Maybe because I had never been exposed to this kind of urban legend I am able to sit back and be more objective than the general public. Maybe it is because I am a Chiropractor and am used to people telling me the most outlandish things for the last fourteen years. Whatever the reason the first time I heard the statement that all I was losing was water weight, I thought it was a joke. The second, third, and fourth time I heard this, I was dumbfounded.

Most people start this argument with "Now I am not a doctor, but".

I happen to be a doctor so I tend to like to think before I speak. We are now going to play a little game called "Lets Think about This". I know that I sound sarcastic but I can't help it. I don't care how many doctors tell you something, it is your job to think. I am quite sure Dr. Atkins had every one of his colleagues telling him that he was wrong and stupid, and would only end up hurting people. Actually they were probably saying much worse and threatening him with the loss of his medical license.

Back to the heart of the argument. The argument is that the first 10 pounds of weight loss is water weight. I am going to be talking about fast's in general and then more specifically about the Fast Diet.

If I stopped eating why would I lose water weight? Did my body all of a sudden stop making ADH (Anti diuretic hormone)? Does my body say to itself, *hey there are no more calories coming in, so let's get rid of the water that we need to maintain our cellular health and our immune and vascular systems?* That makes no sense. If all input stopped, the body would try to conserve all of its resources for as long as possible. I would think that water would be the last thing to be squandered.

Next argument. You stopped eating, so the weight you are losing is water weight. How? We lose water mainly through respiration, sweating, and urination. I have gone long periods between meals in my life for one reason or other, and never once did I break down and lose 10 pounds of sweat. I also didn't overflow the toilet with urine. I know I didn't breath out an extra two gallons of water. So my question remains the same. How?

⚜ ⚜ ⚜

A NOTE TO MY READERS:

The last couple of paragraphs were about if I quit eating. Well I did quit eating, but during a fast, I didn't quit drinking! No one ever started a fast with the intention of not drinking. That is unless you are on some hunger protest and trying to get out of jail or something equally fantastic. I believe that most people who are fasting will increase their consumption of fluids.

This does two things, it helps you feel full and it also partially satisfies the oral fixation needs. Even if your consumption does not increase, there is absolutely no rhyme nor reason for someone to decrease their fluid intake. That just doesn't make sense.

When I was a kid I was on the High School swim team. Everybody, and I mean everybody, knew that they could not go swimming for a half an hour after they ate or they would get cramps. I myself knew this to be a fact, because I had been told by my parents, my teachers, the doctors, TV, and my swim coach. However at least once a week on my way to swim practice, I would stop in some fast food place and grab a burger, fries, and a soda. Many a time I would sit in the parking lot finishing off my burger or fries before walking to the pool. Not once did I get a cramp. This wasn't splashing in the shallow end of the swimming pool either; this was for conditioning and competition.

Enough of memory lane. My point is that even though I must have eaten hundreds of times just before swimming Never having had a cramp, I still believed that I would get one if I didn't wait one half hour.

I don't know how this water weight loss started, but I must admit that I am curious. I believe that, like I stated before, most people actually increase their fluid intake during a fast. This will increase renal activity, and cause excessive urination. Although the volume expelled is much greater than normal, the volume intake is increased as well. There should be no net loss of fluids allowing the cells and tissue fluids to remain Isotonic.

With the Fast Diet, the statement of 10 pounds of lost water weight is doubly absurd. The Fast Diet is not a true fast by definition. You are eating the whole time you are fasting. Because you are eating there is no reason for the body to shut down and try to hoard. With the Fast Diet your food consumption is melons. I have not taken the effort to find out how much water is in a bite of Melon. I can tell you, it is a lot. They don't call it *Water*melon for nothing. I can state for an unequivocal fact, that after eating one half of a melon you have consumed large quantities of water. I dare say that you better not be driving in a car right after eating that much melon, if you are be prepared to pull over frequently. If that is not an option you will learn the hard way how much water is in a melon.

Let's recap this a little bit. First, with the Fast Diet, you are eating melons. Melons are loaded with water. It doesn't matter what kind of melon, they all have a great deal of water in them. I know that some melons have more water than others, and some even act as a diuretic, but every one has high water content. Second I also state in the Fast Diet plan that I get a large 32 oz. tea in the morning and drink it during the day. I do this every day. I also drink yogurt, and have a hot tea or two at night. I have an occasional glass of milk, or if I am feeling really frisky, I might have a glass of unfiltered apple juice. The point is, that during this period my fluid intake is through the roof. Their is no reason for my weight loss to be from body fluids, if anything it should cause me to retain the weight..

Let's look for the silver lining. When you do your own fast, learn from my mistakes. Any weight gain that occurs when you are trying to lose, is catastrophic to your desire to continue. If you are like me, the first thing I think of is, "lets just quit, it is not working any way". So when you come to your eat-day during the Fast Diet, approach it with some decorum and a salad fork. Not two open hands and a feeding trough like I did.

Friday, February 27th,

Glorious day today. The scale is now my dearest friend instead of my implacable enemy. I lost another 2 pounds yesterday. Actually it was a pound and 3/4 but I am not going to split hairs. I figure if I was naked it would be 2 pounds, so 2 pounds it is. I am now down to 222 pounds. My record in recent memory is 223 pounds. So, much like the stock market, I have plunged to the lows of the 1990's. I had more watermelon and yogurt today and about a 1/8 of a papaya. I threw in the papaya just to kind of shake things up. Also since I am doing this in the winter, it is hard to find good ripe melons. Papaya is also loaded with vitamins and enzymes, just in case I am running low on anything.

Once again, I almost cracked during the 7 till 9 hour timeframe. This time period is so hard for me. I thought it would get easier but it hasn't. It may just be that recently my wife has been fixing the kids some of my favorites. The felon last night was _pancakes_. Pancakes, why not whip up some homemade cheesecake along with it. I have even begun to try and persuade my kids to just have a salad for supper.

As you can imagine that is going over like a lead balloon. I really am going to make everybody eat something mundane like soup, just to see if it is the food or the habit of eating during that time frame that is the culprit.

My wife told me today that I weighed 215 lbs. when we were married fourteen years ago. She told me that she remembered because two months before the wedding I was knocking myself out getting back into shape. I don't know if this is true, since I have no memory of my life before marriage. However I will take it as a fact.

My original plan was to do the Fast Diet for two weeks and see what happened. I originally only hoped to break the 220 pound barrier and be back in the teens. I know some of you skinny people who are reading this because you just want to fit into a dress or have to make weight for some kind of competition are thinking, "well that is still fat". In my case I would have to agree with you. However it is not _as_ fat.

Just to show you how the world works, I was bragging about my latest 2 pounds - feeling great and the first thing the person said was, "Isn't that all just water weight"? NO! How much water can I possibly be losing? I have lost 11 pounds after seven days on the Fast Diet. I would have lost even more if it wasn't for my two days of gluttony.

My caloric intake has been reduced to almost nothing. I know it is a stretch of the imagination, but couldn't that be why I am losing weight. What is the old saying? "Move more, eat less." I am certainly not moving more but I am eating less. It is not water I am losing, it is fat. I have yet to wake up in a puddle of water with my pillow and sheets soaking wet, (well maybe a couple of times in college after a righteous party, but I don't think it was water). The Fast Diet is not even a true diet. It is only a vehicle to lose weight healthily, easily, and quickly. The Fast Diet was never intended to be a long term change in my eating habits.

Some people take joy watching a sunset, others by watching kids play. Me - I take joy in watching the scale go down and making up new goals just so I can watch the pounds tumble.

I had another pleasant surprise today. Since it is the half-way point of my Fast Diet, I decided to take my blood pressure again. It was 3:00 p.m. when I took it so it would be close enough to the same time I had originally measured it. I had my doubts about taking it now, since the kids and wife were here with me at the office. The other car is in the shop getting repaired. I decided that this would be a fair test of the effects of the fast. This was a truer test of my daily life than just lying on a couch and contemplating my navel.

The results are in and my blood pressure was down to 117/78. I can't ever remember it being that low. I wish I had thought to take my cholesterol reading at the beginning of the fast. I have no proof, but I am willing to bet that it has dropped a great deal as well. I can't even take it now since I have no idea what it was before. All in all I have had more pleasant surprises than bad ones. Now I also get to look forward to checking my blood pressure, just one more little spark of hope and joy in a mundane life.

I have mentioned that I was having a great deal of excess energy lately. I have tried scrupulously to refrain from exercising.

I am still doing that but in all honesty my current level of inactivity is much greater than normal. It is almost as hard not going out bike riding or golfing as it is not eating between the seven and nine witching hours. That is why I hope to be forgiven when I admit that I went for five laps on the treadmill yesterday. I didn't run, I only walked them at a moderate pace but it still burned about 70 calories. So you purists need to keep that in mind when you do your own fast/diet.

Saturday, February 28.

Today was kind of surprising and disappointing. Yesterday I began eating papaya instead of melon. I also decided to give myself a treat and opened a can of chicken noodle soup. I diluted the broth and gave all of the chicken and noodles to my kid. It tasted great. I drank as much broth as I could hold; just for the warm fuzzy feeling it gave me, as well as the change of taste. The soup broth and the papaya made for quite the festive day at my house. It also sent me to the bathroom for the first time in a couple of days. There must be a world of difference between a papaya and a melon.

I weighed today. I am now down to 221 ½. The old me would have been ecstatic over losing a half of a pound. The new me sits on the edge of depression. Like I said before, I am easily discouraged in the weight loss world. I will have to see if I can find out if there is anything special in the papaya that has prevented me from losing as much weight as I have become accustomed to.

I believe I have figured out why the weight loss was only a half pound instead of the one and a half pound average I have been enjoying. The papaya is a much denser fiber food and it takes longer to break down and be processed. The melon is so fluid that the water passes right through within a couple of hours. The amount of organic matter left behind from a melon is really pretty insignificant. If I am correct tomorrow or the next day I should see a jump in the weight loss again. Whether I am right or wrong about the jump in weight loss, I think I am going to have to take papaya off of the list of approved foods for the Fast Diet. It is just too dense and falls in the fruit family instead of the melon family. Like grandmother said, "you can't mix apples and oranges."

Unfortunately I am not going to be able to test this theory of the papaya this time around. Today is scheduled to be an eat day for me. So it will nullify whether I have retained the papaya or not.

Talk about mixed emotions! On the one hand I am giddy with excitement that I can eat whatever I want today. On the other hand I am terrified, because I can eat whatever I want today. Let us not forget what happened last time I was allowed to eat. Can we all say Glutton? Last time I felt like a sailor on shore leave in Bangkok. This time I hope to act more like the sailor who is hung over and broke.

Although I fully expect a set back after eating today, I still feel these little breaks are essential to being able to stick with the fast. The first day of a fast is by far the hardest. The first day allows you to tell yourself things like "lets go ahead and eat today too, we will start fasting tomorrow." In my case I am worse than that. I tell myself things like, "…eat everything you can, because after tonight you get nothing". The point is it doesn't matter if it is a new job or a household project, starting something is the hardest part. Trust me on this people, I am not criticizing when I say quit making excuses. I am by far the worst one out there when it comes to finally getting around to doing things. My wife's honey-do list is only two items long. Even she has finally given up on getting me to start things. I think the only reason I still get a list is for appearance sake.

❦ ❦ ❦

A NOTE TO MY READERS:

Inertia. We have to talk about inertia. Inertia as it applies to the Fast Diet is the forward energy of something over time. No I am not trying to turn everyone into physicists. I am just trying to explain why some of you will have more trouble than others starting and maintaining your Fast. As I stated previously, I have been fat for a decade. I gained 20 pounds with my first kid, and lost 5. I gained 20 pounds with my second kid, and lost 5 again. That is a total of 40 pounds gained and 10 pounds lost, giving me a net gain of 30 pounds. It has fluctuated some over the years, but has pretty much held steady at the 30 pound level. This is not an excuse or a plea for forgiveness for being fat. The point is this, that for ten years I have been happily sailing along at a certain weight. For me to all of a sudden decide, "Hey let's lose 20 or 30 pounds," was really difficult for me. I had no stimulus for doing so. I had no illicit rendezvous with an old flame coming to town, high school reunion, or if you can believe it not even any model shoots scheduled. The fact is I really don't know what caused me to attempt my fast. To make it even worse was that I wasn't sure that I would be able to stick with it for more than a day, even before I began. I was doomed to failure before I even started.

There are a million reasons to *not* do something. It doesn't matter if they are good reasons or bad ones. The fact of the matter is, that it is simply easier not to do something, than it is to do it. I have wanted to lose weight for as long as I can remember. Even when I wasn't fat, I thought I was. It is safe to say that almost my entire life, I have wanted to do something about it. When I was younger, it was no problem, I just played more. After adulthood set in, and especially after I became a parent, the desire to lose weight, took a back seat to raising the kids. Not only did I not do anything about it, but those became my primo weight gaining years. I still wanted to lose weight, but now I had even more excuses not to. Now I could blame the kids and the goodies that they require for my weight. All in all I had a new endless supply of excuses not to do something.

Folks, this is a hard fact of reality. No matter what we tell ourselves, be it a thyroid problem, big boned, muscle weighs more than fat, or even genetics, they are all just excuses. It doesn't matter if you are totally encased in cement, except for your head and neck, if you are the one who is opening and closing your mouth, you have no excuse to not lose weight.

Let me stress, this is not a criticism. In all honesty I would give myself the 'muscle-weighs-more-than-fat' excuse. I even believed it. The only thing holding us back is inertia. We have been at a standstill or worse, moving in the other direction for to long. Now a tremendous amount of effort has to be made to break the suction of inertia, and allow us to rise above it. For those that have been traveling away from their goal they must now stop and then reverse their forward momentum.

Whatever you can latch onto to break your current state of inertia, do it. Grab hold like the proverbial drowning man and his twig. If you don't have a real reason such as a special event, make one up. I am serious; convince yourself that if you don't lose a certain amount of weight, by a certain day you might not be around anymore. Whatever it takes to get started - do it. This bears repeating, doing nothing is easy, doing something is *hard*! Once you manage to start the Fast Diet, momentum will now begin to work for you. Unlike most diets, with the Fast Diet, you don't have to wait weeks to see results. You will see significant results within days. It is a beautiful thing when the scale changes from being your hated enemy, to your beloved friend.

It is like "NIKE" says, "JUST DO IT".

One of my character strengths is that I am impetuous. Some may see this as a negative; I personally see it as a positive. I was watching some movie or television show, when one of the actors said something about a fast. Now I am not sure what was different about that night and all of the other times I have heard the word 'fast,' but something was. It clicked and I decided that, that was what I would do. Now I was left with the *how* of the matter. A fast is simple. Don't eat. Done, said, no more. The reality of a fast is much harder. No one tells you about all of the psychological, visual, olfactory, and taste withdrawals you will experience. These are not to be ignored, these are the things that will make or break your ability to continue on a successful fast.

Sunday, March 1

Today I was not able to get to the office till the afternoon. Anybody that has kids knows that some days your plans just don't really seem to matter. The reason that I mention this is that my scale is at my office. I have been weighing at 9:00 a.m. every day of the fast. It is now four o'clock in the afternoon. I must stress that when you are doing your own fast, it is imperative that you try and weigh at the same time every day. Depending on how much melon or fluid you drink throughout the day your weight could be up to two, even 3 pounds different from when you wake up. A great example of that is what I have done today. I woke up and had a one quarter of a watermelon, and a glass of milk. Since then I have also had lunch consisting of honeydew, and cantaloupe. I have also had a 32 oz tea, yogurt, and various other glasses of fluids to quench my thirst. Granted some of this has been processed and left the body, but the tea alone is 2 pounds of weight. I have no idea how much weight was in the watermelon and cantaloupe, to say nothing about the glasses of liquid I have drunk.

I am now up to 223 ½ pounds. I expected to be heavier today as Saturday was an eat day for me. I am really kind of disappointed that today of all days I was unable to get to the office and weigh. Now my results are really skewed. I don't know how much of the weight gain is from Saturday or from what I have eaten so far on Sunday.

Saturday I did really well all morning long. I had six slices of bacon and that was it. I took the family to a "u-pick" strawberry field and ate myself silly. They were at the peak of ripeness, and who really cares about a little bug poison on the berries. It was like when I was a little kid - one for the bucket, two for me. Eventually the bucket was full and we left. I then stopped off at another fruit stand to load up on melons. Still doing well and holding strong, until my daughter walks up with a fresh baked loaf of banana nut bread, and regular banana bread. Then the fatal words game out of her mouth, "Dad I can't make up my mind so can I get both"? That started my downfall. I still had not been going crazy like I did last time I had an eat day, but I had been yearning for a steak all day.

Parenting being what it is and kids being what they are I never was able to get my steak. So I settled for a big three inch wide slice of banana nut bread with butter. I later had a bowl of Chili with cheese and various nuts and chips as I walked around the house. All and all it wasn't really a bad day of eating.

I did mention that I had wanted a steak today and with me, an unfulfilled desire, eventually turns into an itch. So even though I wasn't hungry I still was looking for something that would just hit the spot. Ironically I was being good when I got into trouble. I was moving around some of the fruit seeing which kind I wanted when I saw a baggie with something in it. Low and behold it was a big piece of leftover steak.

It is now about eleven o'clock in the evening and I have a date with the sand man soon. As soon as I saw that meat, out it came and into the frying pan. I don't even think there was a conscious connection between my brain and my hand. I just woke up and there it was cooking away. The irony of the whole matter is, that by the time I found the steak I wasn't remotely hungry. As a matter of fact I was unable to even finish the steak, and gave the rest to the dog.

ॐ ॐ ॐ

A NOTE TO MY READERS:

The point to be learned here is that I am a horrible example to follow. If you want this fast to work you must have in your mind a goal. My only goal was to do this for two weeks. I have found that this is *not* enough. With a time frame for a goal you are not motivated enough. For example, if I had to weigh a certain amount to be hired for a job as a flight attendant, I would not binge as much and eat smarter on my 'eat' days. I might not even eat as much melon as I do now. If I have a set weight to attain then my motivation would be the less I take in the quicker I reach my goal. With that kind of thought process you are much less likely to binge and give in to any visual stimulus for food.

Now let's look at it from my approach. I took this on for numerous reasons. First, and foremost, was to lose weight. Second was a curiosity about my own willpower and my ability to see this through to the end. Third was that as a Doctor, I had my own theories and ideas about health and weight loss that I wanted to explore.

All of these are good and valid reasons for me attempting and sticking with my fast. But none of them were great reasons. A great reason is a wedding in two weeks; a boxer having a weigh-in; or meeting a weight requirement for a job. Those are all great reasons. Those are do or die scenarios. When you compare those reasons against mine you can also see the goal will be much easier to attain with a great reason. Since I didn't have a great reason for sticking to the plan I had to come up with something else. What I came up with was brevity. If I had a reward just a few days away, I could stick with the Fast Diet plan. That is why the beginning of the Fast is only 3 days.

The three days of fasting with a break afterwards is very important to those of us who need encouragement. There is a powerful psychological advantage to the set up of this plan. Day one you are all fired up, and fast with good spirits, ignoring cookies like they were not even there. Day two you wake up and go to work. By the time you start thinking about food it is already lunch time. You may be getting hit now with visual temptations as well as the habit to eat at noon. Instead of giving in and snacking, or quitting, you just have to realize that after tomorrow I can eat again. By doing this you are already past the halfway point to where you can eat again. This is very simple yet extremely powerful for people like me who need the motivation to stay the course. Those with exceptional powers of observation have realized that I started my weight loss program on a Wednesday. Yes this is a weird day to begin any kind of long term project. Although this seems weird it was done with a reason. Most people would have started something like this on Monday.

My logic for starting this program on Wednesday reflects my lack of willpower. I mentioned before that I have Tuesdays off. I know myself very well. If I had started this plan on Monday, I would have been hanging around the house all day Tuesday with nothing to do but think about the fact that I was not eating. The chances of me sticking with my plan for even two days would have been remote. By starting on Wednesday I had three days where I knew that I would be at work with no temptation to eat. By the time Saturday rolled around I would be able to eat again. If you choose to start your plan on any other day than Wednesday, you need to keep that in mind also.

I will mention this over and over throughout this book. I am nothing special. I am just like you. I may have more guilt about being fat, since I am a college professor as well as a doctor. I have no excuse, not only should I know better, I do know better than to over eat. Then again millions of doctors and college professor's smoke, what is their excuse?

Back to my point. Having seen thousands of ads about 'take this pill lose this weight,' or 'join this program to lose the weight,' etc., I admit to being tempted a time or two, to buy some of those pills and things. I even have a dark confession to make. Once I joined one of those plans where the food is delivered to your house. I must hang my head in shame. I was only able to stick with it for about a week, before I quit. I still have the food. It is in the garage just waiting for the next hurricane to blow through. Just to rub salt in the wound, I didn't realize that it was an automatic renewal plan, and now have two months worth of food. Like I said, the next time a hurricane hits I will be well prepared. I think that stuff has a longer shelf life than the MRE's (Meal Ready to Eat), we got in the army.

Let's look at some of the reasons that this plan did not work for me. I specify for *me*, because every plan works for someone. The first reason is that I fell for a slick advertising campaign. The food on the TV sure looked good, but a more profound reason was that I put the responsibility of me losing weight into the hands of someone else. After all I paid my money for their food, so they should make me lose the weight. If I didn't lose the weight, well that is their fault not mine, afterall, I did what I was supposed to - I bought the food. The stupid diet plan just doesn't work.

The placing of blame and relying on others to insure your success is a trap. If we don't accept the fact that the only reason we are overweight is because of our own actions, we have no chance of succeeding. Once we realize this the flip side is a lot more palatable. If we have the power to cause the problem, we also have the power to correct the problem. This is one of the reasons that the Fast Diet plan is so successful. You are the master of your own destiny. There is no volume limits, to this plan, there is no measuring, and there is no guessing about portion size. This plan is simplicity itself. If you feel like eating a half a melon, go ahead. If you feel like only eating a bite or two, that's also fine.

One of the main drawbacks to conventional diet plans is exactly that, they are planned. The problem with that is that, what is more than satisfying for one person will leave another grossly disappointed and unfulfilled. Measured portions cause a number of problems. The first is that it is measured. I don't like to take the time to act like a scientist in the kitchen. I don't want all of my beakers and scales, just so I can fill up my bowl with cereal. If something is measured, you are going to be like Goldilocks and the three bears. This one is too much, this one is too little, and maybe, this one is just right. It is all unnecessary. Those plans leave you with a feeling of guilt. It happens like this, I already have my 3ozs of protein but I really want more. Do you or don't you? Do you take the three ounces and walk away feeling unsatisfied? Or do you add some more protein and walk away feeling guilty that you are cheating on your diet?

You should say this out loud when you begin to falter, Cheating leads to Quitting.

However you look at it, it is always the same. The simplest things work the best. I am not going to go point by point in critiquing a planned diet vs. the Fast Diet. All of us have seen planned diets before. Just picture in your mind which method you would find easier to live with. The Fast Diet is unplanned. It has a stringent outline, but whatever you do within those guidelines is up to you.

Let's look at a typical day on the Fast Diet. You wake up and are running late for work. You don't even have time for a bite of melon, because you forgot to cut one up last night. You just jump in your car and go to work. I am sure that you have done this a thousand times before. There is no penalty for this. No one is going to yell at you because you missed your 8:30 feeding time. When you get home for lunch, you are not only allowed 'X' number of ounces, eat until you are full, but if you can't decide between honeydew and watermelon, eat them both. If you are still kind of full from lunch and don't feel like supper, fine, skip it. Go make yourself a hot tea with milk and honey and curl up in front of the television. If you get hungry later, no problem, eat some more melon.

This plan allows you the freedom to live your life without being a slave to some prepared plan that you had no chance to give your input into.

Monday March 2

This is a pivotal day for me. Saturday was my last scheduled eat day. Sunday as I stated earlier I had gained some weight as expected but I didn't know if it was from all of the food, or because I was not able to weigh until the afternoon. As silly as it seems, I was greatly concerned over the possibility that it was all food.

I stepped on the scale today and am back down to, 222. That is still one half pound heavier than I went into the weekend weighing, but still not nearly as devastating as my original eat days.

I am coming into the home stretch now. I only have three more days of the Fast Diet left. By now I would have expected to be tired and waiting with baited breath for the end of this thing. Instead I am more like a racer who sees he has a chance to break a world record. Now, I am not hungry in the slightest, nor do I have any real desire to quit. During my final sprint, I think that I might even cut back on the amount of melon I eat. Sunday I ate a whole medium sized water melon. I didn't really want to, but it was a cold rainy day and I was stuck at home with nothing to do. I find this fact pleasant but hard to believe, I still really like eating melon. This makes sticking with the plan much easier.

Now that I am this close to the end I have found that my goals have changed. Testing my willpower and scientific curiosity are now out the window. I know that I can go the distance with the Fast Diet.. It doesn't matter f I quit now or after next Wednesday. My theories and ideas about losing weight in an unconventional manner have been proven more effective than I ever hoped. Now it is 100% about losing weight. I really wanted to get down to the two hundred and teens. That would have made my decade. I haven't been below 220 in over ten years. Now my goal is to get to 215. That is my marriage weight and something that I never expected to see again.

Tuesday, March 3,

I lost a pound yesterday and am now down to 221 lbs. Once again I am back in the black. There is nothing ahead of me except uncharted weight loss. Every ounce I lose from this point on will be a new record of skinny for me.

I now know what a bi-polar person feels like. One minute I am on cloud nine because I am going to break the 220 barrier, the next I am depressed because I won't make my marriage weight. There is also the added distraction of the end of the diet arriving with all of the rewards that implies.

ॐ ॐ ॐ

A NOTE TO MY READERS:

Let me try to explain some of the things that I am currently feeling. I will try to cover these feelings in order. First let's talk about the weight loss. Even after the gains I experienced over the first and second eating periods I have still lost about 12 pounds. Twelve pounds in less than two weeks, (Are You Kidding Me??), I should be running around kissing babies. Instead all that I can think of is, if I hadn't taken the time off and eaten on those two occasions, I would be about 6 to 7 pounds lighter. If I had done it that way not only would I have made my marriage weight goal of 215, but I would already be below it, and well on my way to being in the single digits. Instead of being excited I am actually leaning toward the depressed spectrum. I realize that this is foolish but it cannot be helped. Unfortunately for me, when I think this way it is a *very* easy step for me to quit. My thought process tends to go something like this: "Well I won't reach my goal, so I have already lost. I might as well quit now, there is no reason to keep going just to say I finished".

To counteract this thought process, I must remind myself that my original goal was to do this plan for two weeks. There was no amount of weight mentioned, no marriage weight, no getting below 220, nothing. The only reason that I am feeling depressed at all is that the plan worked so well it allowed me to start dreaming about levels that I thought were gone for ever.

Let's talk about the 6 to 7 pounds I gained and again lost during this plan. Yes they make me mad, yes they infuriate me, and yes they even kind of embarrass me. I wish with all of my heart that I did not gain those extra pounds during this two week period. I want to make sure that there is no ambiguity about my feelings when it comes to the weight gains during my plan.

Now, it is time to hear the hard brutal truth. I could not have completed this plan without those breaks built into it. There was no way I could have gone two weeks without quitting. I would have started slowly cheating, and then cheating fast, and then wake up one day with a mouthful of bacon. It would have been so gradual that I would not have even realized that I quit, until my wife or kids would ask me how my diet was going. So for me and people like me, those breaks in the plan are 100% necessary. If I didn't lose as much as I could have, so be it. If they were not there, would I have lost a great deal more weight? No. Because I would have quit.

If you are of strong will you might not need those breaks. I am just not in that league. I strongly recommend that you take the breaks to put a little extra protein in your system and prevent plateauing on your diet.

I also mentioned that the end of the plan looming closer is causing me problems. This is really not as big a problem as the weight gain, but it still comes into play. Because the end is so near I am beginning to tell myself that since I won't make my goal, just quit. I know I stated this before, but I want to clarify something for you. When you are doing this plan there should be no end-of-plan confusion.

I said at the beginning that I tied my hands when I began this plan; that I was doing it for two weeks as well as cutting out exercise. When you are doing your own Fast Diet, there is no reason for you to put a rock solid time frame into your plan. If you have a goal and you are a pound or two away from it, feel free to extend your fast. Not only that, if you need to accelerate the plan, incorporate exercise into your plan. The only reason that I have not exercised, is that I absolutely didn't want to have to rely on increased exercise to achieve my desired results. Against all odds this plan does exactly that, it does not rely on exercise to achieve results.

This program came about because I had certain ideas that the rest of the "knowledgeable" people disagreed with. So I had to approach this in a scientific manner. I had to decrease the variables such as exercise and duration. That was done specifically for data, *not results*. The fantastic results that I experienced were achieved in spite of, not because of, the limits I put on myself.

I so wish Dr. Atkins was still alive. I would give him a big hug, and say "brother I feel your pain." Then we would sit down and talk about how infuriating and difficult it is to buck the system when you know you are right.

Wednesday, March 4,

This is my last day on the Fast Diet. I gave myself a heart attack today. I came in to weigh, like I do every morning at 9:00 a.m., but when I stepped on the scale - it didn't move. Not only did it not move but it showed I gained about a 1/4 pound. I had a bad couple of minutes there, until I remembered that the day before I set my scale forward to how much I thought I would lose by today. It turns out I was a little optimistic. I anticipated (*hoped*), I would lose a pound and 1/4, on Tuesday. I didn't lose that much but I did lose a pound.

In retrospect, I think it was a minor miracle that I was able to lose a pound or even an ounce today. I swear, whenever we try something that will improve our situation, the world will conspire to prevent that from happening.

I have mentioned previously that I have two kids. I have a little eight year old boy named Conner and a little ten year old girl named Hunter. Conner is not the problem. He wants to be waited on hand and foot when it comes to eating. So he is pretty much at our mercy regarding what he gets to eat. Hunter, on the other hand, is learning how to cook. Not only is she learning how to cook, she is also learning how to bake. Let me reiterate, it is Tuesday afternoon, I have one day left of my Fast Diet. It is my day off so I do not have the refuge of the office to keep me away from any and all stimulus for eating. Even if I did have that stimulus, my brain has been trained for the last fourteen years that there is nothing to eat there.

Instead I am at home pacing the house like a caged tiger. My head is a jumble of conflicting emotions. Will I break 220? If I don't break 220 do I consider myself a failure? Should I stop it now and have just one little bite? All of these things have been going throughout my brain all day long. Against all odds, I held strong. Then I was thrown into Dante's 7th level of hell. My lovely little daughter, decided she wanted to try and make (all by herself), a pan of homemade chocolate brownies. We haven't made brownies ever; I don't think my wife has ever tried making them. Now, smack dab in my witching hours from 7:00 a.m. to 9:00 a.m., it's cold outside and the whole house smells like fresh baked chocolate brown-ies. I am ashamed to admit that I cracked. Every time I took some body's plate to the kitchen, I ate whatever crumbs were on the plate. My only speck of pride was that I didn't actually take a bite out of a whole brownie.

Now for the most important announcement of the day. I am now sitting dead on 220 pounds. It is very exciting for me, to be at this weight. It is kind of like the second before you say "I do". You know that when you wake up tomorrow, something is going to be different.

⚘ ⚘ ⚘

A NOTE TO MY READERS:

You will be tempted during the plan. You may even break down completely and binge. Or you may be one of those godlike beings, who stare temptation in the face and walk away pure and untarnished. Whatever personality type you are, it really doesn't matter. If you are weak or made of steel, you will meet your goal. That is the beauty of this program. I binged a couple of times during this two week period and yet I still managed to lose more weight than I ever expected.

I meant to talk about this earlier, but forgot until I men-tioned waking up. Starting about the eighth, day of the Fast Diet, I noticed a change in my sleep patterns. Normally I come home about seven o'clock in the evening. If there is any homework still to be done I help the kids with that, take orders from the family, play some with the kids, help a little with dinner, and then yell at the kids to take a shower, brush their teeth, and go to bed. After that it is time with the wife and either television or a book. Because of that schedule I tend to stay up till around 12:30 -1:00 am. When I do go to bed I fall asleep instantly, but tend to wake up off and on throughout the night.

I began to notice that after about day eight of the Fast Diet, I had been having trouble staying awake past 11:00 p.m. I still fall asleep instantly, but now I sleep like a log throughout the night. I consider this to be a huge unforeseen benefit of this plan.

I need to mention this while I am talking about sleep. I learned this the hard way, so there is no need for you to learn it over again. When I first began the Fast Diet, I ate melon right up till the time I went to bed. I did this because I was in the habit of snacking throughout the evening. At first my snacking habit was too strong for me to overcome, so I just substituted the snacks with melon. To my delight, I discovered that my snacking habit decreased dramatically. After all, if you think about it, a snack is just something to either satisfy a hunger or because it tastes good. In my case I wasn't hungry - I was in a rut. My snacks were of the taste-good variety.

Anyone who has kids knows that there are going to be lunch box treats somewhere in the house. All you have to do is know where they are hidden. So my snacking problem was not because I was hungry, it was because I wanted a *"goodie"*.

I did not attempt to change anything with my grazing habits. All I did was substitute the *"goodie"*, with melon. This satisfied my habit of grabbing something from the kitchen every time I went there as well as putting something sweet into my mouth. After a few days my snack cycle went away with barely a whimper. I still go in the kitchen, but the times I look for something to eat have greatly decreased. After awhile the message even penetrated my thick skull and my decades of hard-wired re-enforcement. The new message that my body was getting was something like this. "Yea, I like this, and yea, it's sweet, but I had this for breakfast, lunch, and dinner. I think I will just skip the snack and go back to the living room." Without even realizing it, my trips to the kitchen have almost stopped. I hope that this continues after I am done with the Fast Diet. Truthfully I don't think they will. If they don't, I plan on having a bowl of melon at all times in the fridge. So I can keep re-enforcing my newly laid brain circuitry.

All of this has been leading up to a point that needs to be made. Even though I was sleeping well, all of that fluid I was imbibing was making me get up two or three times a night to go to the bathroom. My kidneys and bladder haven't gotten a work out like this since my college days; the only difference is that I am not waking up with a hangover now. I personally don't drink many fluids. According to everyone I know I should be a raisin by now. I have begun to not eat any more melon after 9:30 p.m.; this seems to work fine for me.

The problem of nocturnal emissions might not be a problem for you, but at the beginning when your body is starting to regulate itself, expect more trips to the bathroom than usual. If you are one of these people who drink three quarts of water a day, you might not notice any change whatsoever. For the rest of us, it is a pretty big adjustment to make and something that needs to be planned for. If you are incontinent I strongly advise against this plan.

Thursday, March 5

I finished my diet plan yesterday. I will get to the important part about how much weight I lost in a minute. Before I get to that, there is something very important that I must discuss. Being *"normal"*, I did something very foolish yesterday. I cheated on myself. To make breaking the 220 mark a slam dunk. I keep trying to justify my stupidity by stating that unlike you, I have a certain time frame I imposed upon myself. You will not be burdened by this like me so you probably won't become a basket-case. Whatever the reason, I decided to do something stupid. I wanted to make it into the two hundred and teens so bad that I skipped supper and breakfast. I didn't want one more ounce in my body than was absolutely necessary. As a result, I found myself getting light headed every time I got up from a chair, or stood up from bending over my patients. Once twelve o'clock noon rolled around and I was able to eat again, my symptoms subsided.

I am glad that this happened to me. As I mentioned before in passing, I read about fasting during my two weeks. I have also gone online to read about what to expect with a fast and some of the pro's and con's, of a true fast. Most of what I've discovered is more in the line of a Zen experience, and becoming one with nature. Some of what the books and online sites speak of are the expected side effects. One of the serious side effects of a *true* Fast is that if you stop eating anything, you will throw off your electrolytes. That can lead to heart palpitations dizziness, weakness, and a host of other undesirable symptoms.

As a physician I already knew what would happen with a drastic change in fluid chemistry. I did not feel like I needed to say anything about this problem, since The Fast Diet, is not a true fast. It is mostly a fast, but never are you completely not eating. The food (melons), that you eat contains stored electrolytes and energy. If you follow the plan you should not ever find yourself in a severe electrolyte deficiency.

If you do begin to get some symptoms of light headedness check your blood pressure first. One of the side effects of the Fast Diet is a lowered blood pressure. In my case this was not really an issue. If you are a person with very high or low blood pressure and you experience a significant drop, your body will go through a period of adjustment. During this period it is quite common to have periods of light headedness. This is good because your body is adapting to a more efficient state.

Time for the drum roll. My final weight is 218 pounds. I didn't reach my Marriage weight of 215, but I did meet all of my other goals. I deem the Fast Diet to be a complete success.

I took my final blood pressure reading today at 3:00 p.m. It is slightly up from last time but still well within the good range. It is 120/80. With only a three point shift, in my systolic pressure and I am not very concerned. I actually thought it would be somewhat higher, since I tweaked my electrolytes this morning. Either it has already reached equilibrium again, or my blood chemistry was not as effected as it seemed. So let's recap:

Let's do some recapping.

Beginning Weight:	233lbs
Eat Period one	+ 4lbs
Eat Period two	+ 2lbs
Total	239lbs
Ending Weight	218lbs
	239LBS
	- 218lbs
Total Weight Lost	21 lbs
Net Weight Lost	15lbs
Time period of Diet Plan	Two Weeks
Actual Days Fasting	12
Average Weight loss per day	1.75lbs

Chapter Two

The Plan – Putting It to the Test

Now, let's review:

DAY 1-3

Only eat melons, and whatever one of the teas, yogurt milk or juices you want to drink

DAY 4-5

Eat and drink whatever you like.

DAY 6-11

Only eat Melons, coffee/teas, yogurt milk, or juices you want to drink; you can also substitute soup broth for two of your meals during this period.

Day 12

Eat and drink whatever you like.

Day 13-15

Only eat melons, coffee/teas, milk, yogurt or juices you want to drink.

On a side note, I did reach my marriage weight of 215 pounds. I stayed on the Fast Diet for an additional four days. The reason it took me so long to go from 218 down to 215, was that since I was technically not on the plan anymore I felt justified in snacking "a little bit." This proves my point – there is no such thing as just a little snacking

I drank a lot of tea during this period of weight loss for two reasons. The first reason was that I like tea, the second was that I needed something completely opposite from a melon, just to let me forget that I was on any kind of diet plan.

I didn't drink coffee because I just don't like it. Coffee is also a diuretic. On the Fast Diet, I spent enough time in the evenings going to the bathroom; I didn't need to do it more. If this doesn't bother you coffee should be fine if you don't put sugar or artificial sweetener in it. The milk I used was 2% organic milk. Whole milk is fine, but has a high caloric fat content. The only sweetener that I used was non-processed honey; if sugar cane juice is available, it is also a good alternative.. You can use whatever kind of sweetener you like as long as it is natural and unprocessed. Everything on the plan should be whole foods that have not been processed. Save your junk for the eat days. I used liquid yogurt as one of my beverages. I also used unfiltered apple juice, and orange juice with pulp, Grapefruit juice, is fine also. If you have a juicer, anything that you can get juice out of will work. The only criteria are that it is natural and unprocessed. I know that I could have lost more weight if I just drank water, but I really don't like drinking plain water.

On two occasions I used soup broth for my supper. I tend to get tired of a cold supper every night. As a matter of fact after the first week I found myself leaving my melons out of the refrigerator, just so they would be at least room temperature.

The soup was fine, but it tends to have a high sodium content that may cause you to retain fluids. Also if you substitute too many of your meals with soup broth the sodium content may became too high for some individuals to tolerate well. Normally this shouldn't be a problem, but it will make you thirsty and possibly cause you to consume more liquid calories than necessary. Again that is fine, you will still lose weight. However this is called the Fast Diet for a reason.

I did try mixing some fruits such as papaya, apple, and pineapple into the plan. I am not sure of the actual reason but I did make a guess earlier as to why I think they were not as appropriate for the plan and why they slowed down the weight loss. If you are going to mix fruit with your plan, do it on a miniscule level. If you feel like eating grapes only eat about five or six, not a whole bunch of them. The same goes for apples, eat a slice or two. Don't eat the whole apple. Pineapple is the same; just eat half of a ring of pineapple, not the whole thing. On a side note if you do eat pineapple, don't eat the canned variety that is packed in juice. Eat fresh pineapple from the produce department. That pre-packaged juice is loaded with sugar.

I think that covers all of the food that I ate on my Fast Diet. I am not going to list all of the junk I ate during my eat days.

I realize that fruits are the same as melons in the minds of most people. But in reality, they *aren't!* If you must have the taste of fruit to get you through the day, drink them. Find pre-packaged whole fruit juices, or make your own. Do not supplement your diet by eating them, it won't hurt you but it will slow down your weight loss. If you absolutely must eat something different I have provided a number of suggestions.

I have broken down the appropriate foods into two categories. The Primary foods are strongly recommended, the secondary foods are marginally tolerated within limits. If you feel the need for another taste, it should be on the secondary list of foods as opposed to a Big Mac.

Primary Foods	Secondary Foods
Watermelon	Grapes
Cantaloupe	Pomegranate
Honeydew melon	Papaya
Musk melon	Pineapple
Christmas melon	Apple
All other Melons	Citrus fruits
	Cucumbers
	Soup broth (maximum 3 xs)

Just so there is no misunderstanding, you can eat all of the primary foods as often and as much as you like. There is no limit. The secondary foods will slow down your weight loss. They will not cause you to gain weight but the secondary foods do have limits.

You should only eat one of the secondary foods when you are just sick to death of melon. As I mentioned before, the secondary foods have more substance to them. This means that your body must use more energy to process and digest the fruit fibers. This process takes away from the main business of breaking down stored energy.

I strongly recommend against using the secondary foods. This plan was set up as a modified fast, with a goal of losing weight in a lightning-like manner. Once you have reached your goal and begin to eat again, you can and should incorporate the secondary foods into your daily routine, try not to do it before.

One of the most important parts of this Plan is the way it is broken down into specific segments and periods of Fasting and eating. Unless you are really, and I mean really good at sticking with things, don't alter the sequence of this plan.

The beginning of the Fast should be three days, If and I mean *if*, you are still jazzed and going strong you can extend the start of the fast portion into Saturday. If you are feeling the slightest cravings don't do it. Take the recommended two days off to eat. Be aware of the temptation to over eat during this first period of eating. If you don't binge and eat sensible, you won't have to re-lose as much as I did.

You should be aware that most people carry pounds of organic matter in their intestinal tract. It can be in the form of an impacted intestinal lining or semi and processed fecal matter. A side benefit of this plan is that it acts as a detoxification and allows your body to deal with some of these issues. If we are not continually pouring more matter in, the body is finally able to clean itself and purge as well as break down the food more completely. The way we do things now, breakfast is still here by the time we start dumping lunch in on top of it. Lunch hasn't even cleared the station before supper arrives. The body is forced to push out the existing food through a peristaltic wave, to make room for the new arrivals. It doesn't matter whether it has been digested or not. It is leaving, and leaving now.

By the time you reach your eat day. You should be pretty hollow and whatever you eat should register on the scale. Don't be discouraged by this weight gain. It isn't like it is layered fat, and should come off as soon as it completes its journey.

Because of what I just stated about the body being able to take longer to fully process the little food you are eating, you will probably find that the interval from mouth to toilet takes longer than you are accustomed to.

After the two days of eating you start a six day period of fasting on the melons again. At the end of this six day period you have another eat day scheduled, don't skip this single eat day. If you do you will suffer burn out. If you don't want to quit your melon intake that is fine but you must eat something that is *not* a melon. This has the double effect of preventing burn out, as well as allowing you to add proteins and fats that you may be lacking.

After the eat day you begin another three days of melon fasting. At the end of this period if you have reached your goal *fantastic!* If not, continue on as if you are doing the six day portion of the melon fast. If at the end of that time you are still not at your desired goal, you should take a few days off and eat sensibly before you begin another two week period on the Fast Diet. Don't instantly start another two weeks without some kind of break. One of the aspects of this plan that makes it quick and very effective is the built in intervals. Every athlete or weight trainer out there will tell you that interval training achieves much greater results than a marathon workout without any breaks built into it.

This experience was also a time of learning for me. I never thought about what I would do once I reached my goal and quit the two week diet plan. It turns out that quitting was not that simple. In the next section of the book I will try and make that transition as simple as possible.

I hope that you are reading this now because you have used the Fast Diet as a vehicle to lose some weight. I also hope that all of your goals have been met or will be met in the near future.

Chapter Three

The Transition – What Happens Next?

We have now gone full circle. We got up from the table, grabbed our own destiny by the horns, and accomplished something great. Congratulations. Now what? When I had met my last goal of getting to my marriage weight, I was suffused with emotions. I did something that I *never* expected to do. I rolled back the clock fifteen years. I was very proud of myself, and I had every right to be proud. I have heard some people say that losing weight was harder than quitting smoking. I don't smoke but I certainly believe them.

Once I met my final goal I was faced with some decisions. The most obvious of them was to just set another goal and keep on trucking. I could have easily told myself we have come this far, let's get into the two hundred and single digits range. Once I hit two hundred and nine, I could have then said let's try and break 200.

I know that you are now on the edge of your seat as to what I decided. Well I will tell you but before I do, I want each and every one of you to try and put yourself into my shoes. I want you to decide for yourselves what you would have done, before you find out what I did.

Remember, I have the will power of a wet noodle. I did not have a great reason for beginning this plan. To make matters worse there was no plan when I began, so unlike you

I had no idea of what to expect or even if what I was doing was going to work. What I did have was a bunch of mediocre reasons that I was able to lump together and manage to draw enough inspiration from to allow me to begin. I will say this over and over, starting is the hardest part.

When I began I set myself an arbitrary deadline at two weeks. I didn't quite just pull that number out of my hat, but it was close. I then took on this project as more of a bet with myself that would allow me to test myself against the conventional wisdom of the ages. It was not until a couple of days into the plan that I actually began to set any weight loss goals for myself. In the beginning I was just going to do it for two weeks and be done. As the plan progressed and my weight began to come off I began to get excited enough to start setting milestones for myself. The weight loss goal was therefore a secondary goal.

I have made no bones about it, I am lacking in will power and motivation to lose another fifteen pounds at this point. Lets face it – losing weight is not fun. In this case it was much less painful than normal, but still it is not fun. This plan was never set up for long term life style changes. It was simply a vehicle for me and others to lose weight in as quick, healthy, and easy a manner as possible. I want to be able to look at a melon as desert again instead of supper.

I hope I don't disillusion you, but I stopped. Yep, I did not go on to break 200 pounds.

What I did was what I always do. I rationalized myself into feeling good about quitting. Unfortunately this is really quite easy for me to do.

By now I am feeling like the Guru of all knowledge as to anything to do with weight loss. I am on cloud nine. I proved my approach to weight loss, I disproved some commonly held beliefs and dogma, and last and most important, I reached my goal of weighing the same now as I did when I was married. I could have used that as my excuse to quit, but I didn't – I got even more creative.

I mentioned earlier at the start of the book that I was a few months shy of 50. Well I am even closer to 50 now. The reason I bring this up is that it plays heavily into my derailment.

I am blessed with a lot of knowledge of anatomy, cellular structure and nutrition and aging. It is said that a little knowledge is dangerous, well a lot of knowledge can be nuclear. This is how I talked myself into quitting.

I am very aware of the effects of aging on the skin. The skin loses its elasticity or ability to shrink after stretching. This ability is further decreased with sun and wind damage over long periods of time. Also if your body is not properly hydrated you will also decrease the stretch factor in your skin.

I am a blond blue eyed Florida kid. I grew up in south Florida on the coast, and spent all of my waking hours in the sun. I am also a surfer, and still surf today. To say my skin has been weathered is an understatement.

When I was a teenager they had not invented sunscreen, I remember many a weekend sitting on the beach with the gang from high school, me with my surfboard and the girls putting baby oil all over themselves for that pretty *"healthy"* tan they all craved. The only sun protection they had at the time was zinc oxide. For those who don't know what that is, it is the same white cream you put on your baby's butt to prevent diaper rash. There was no way a teenage boy was going to walk around looking like a mime. I would not have done that even if we knew the sun was bad for me.

I mention my fun filled youth for a reason. I am very aware of what category my skin condition is in. When I was losing my weight I was paranoid that I would look like a popped balloon. It was all I could think about. Before I lost weight I had a lot of what I termed *"hard fat"*. This is the kind of fat that a retired football player gets. They are overweight but still have a lot of muscle under the fat. That is the category that I put myself in.

Because I surf, I still have pretty big arms and a lot of upper body strength. The additional blubber suit I have worn for the last decade helps keeps me warm and gives me the appearance of being *"big"*, instead of flabby. Once I began to lose weight so quickly, I became obsessive over how lose my skin was becoming. I would walk around constantly pinching my biceps to see how much skin I could get between my fingers. I would also poke myself in the love handles to see if they shook or not. I would have my son and daughter see if they could wrap their hands around my arms and see if they could touch their fingers. Finally I would jump up and down in front of the mirror to judge my jiggle factor (Thank god this is a book and not a movie). Eventually I decided that all of these factors had reached a crisis, and if I went one day longer I would look like a kid wearing his daddy's shirt. In reality not one person ever said a word about me looking like a flying squirrel. I had even gone surfing a few times and still no comment. Believe me when I tell you if it was noticed with that group of guys there would have been lots of comments!

The reality was this. I was thinner, my arms were smaller, my waist was smaller – everything about me was smaller. That was the point of the whole diet. Because of the weight loss my skin was not as tight. However it was not flapping like a wind sock either. But that was my excuse for quitting. I told myself that I would hang out at this weight for a couple of months to allow my skin to shrink back and then do it again.

Now the miracle happened. I finally did get on the scale again two months after I quit my diet plan. Wonder of wonders, the scale read 218 lbs. As neurotic as I am, I had convinced myself that I had regained all of my weight by now. I was ecstatic that I had managed to not gain any weight back. Not only did I feel skinny again, but I was happy to prove another of my theories.

My core belief has always been that if I have been steady at my weight of 235, for a few years, it stood to reason that I could remain steady at a lesser weight also. All I had to do was to lose the weight and get there. That is another reason why I developed my diet plan in the first place. I wanted to reach another plateau and stay there. I didn't want to change my life, or give up things that I liked.

I have not worked very hard, but I have worked at keeping the weight off. I didn't just go back to chips and pizza. What I did was about two days a week I would just have supper. During those two days my breakfast and lunch were melons.

Since I normally don't eat breakfast, that usually just meant that two days I would have melon for lunch. I would also pick one or two days a month and eat nothing but the melon. I still drink unsweetened iced tea instead of sweet tea, but other than that, nothing much has changed in my dietary habits. I will try and substitute melon for candy or ice cream when I have the cravings for something sweet. but even then I am not always successful and will treat myself to some chocolate or ice cream.

One of the things that I noticed was that when I lost my first 20 pounds. I felt diminished. Not weaker, but just less of a presence. I didn't even realize it at the time, but I liked being a presence in a room full of people. I liked being described as the "Big Blond Guy". Don't get me wrong, I am still six feet tall and over two hundred pounds. Unfortunately go to any high school in America and you will see a ton of kids just as tall and just as fat. So even though it was my plan all along I kind of miss the subdued caution I used to command when I walked into a room.

Ah, well, since I was always a lover not a fighter, I will just have to get reacquainted with my roots, and get noticed for my girlish figure instead of being the ogre in the corner.

I will say this – Starting this the second time was much harder than starting it the first time. My motivation just wasn't there. I am 20 pounds lighter, I feel good, my pants don't hurt anymore, and I think I am a babe magnet again. Why would I want to do this all over again? The answer is painfully simple. I don't!

Remember how I told you at the beginning of the book that my motivation was good but not great? This time my motivation was not even good. That is the real reason that I took two months off. (I can be honest with myself now that it is over). It wasn't to let my skin shrink back to my diminished body; I simply didn't want to do it again. Let me restate that. I wanted to lose more weight, but not enough to actually get off the couch and do it.

That is why when I finally did get the courage to weigh myself again I was so excited. All that previous work was not wasted. I also knew that it was now or never. I took every crumb of excitement and motivation I could scrounge off the floor and rolled it into a mass that was just, and I mean *just*, big enough to get me off the couch for round two. I am not going to kid you, sticking with it again was much harder than when I did it the first time. I don't make any apologies; I am just not that much of a self motivator when it comes to losing weight.

I have said this before – it doesn't matter what you do to find the motivation to begin the Fast Diet, but if you feel even the slightest urge to start it, go directly to the farmers market and load up on melons. There is never going to be a better time to start than right this second. I don't care if tomorrow is Thanksgiving. If you have the motivation to start do it *now!* If you don't you will be like me and your start will be ten years down the road.

It doesn't even matter if you quit after a day, the next time you feel the tingle to try it again do it.

I wasn't sure I was going to admit this but 'in for a penny in for a pound.' I myself had about four false starts before I was able to get back on the plan for an extended period again after I reached my goal of 215.. I would start it for a day and that night tell myself, what the heck I will eat steak with the family tonight and start again tomorrow. Or I would go a day or two and the next day would be the weekend. Now I am faced with the entire day of doing stuff with my kids, feeding them watching them run down the ice cream truck, gnawing on a fried chicken leg, etc. I think you get the picture. The easiest thing in the world is to throw in the towel, reach into the bucket, and join the kids at the table. My conscience is clear; my inner voice assures me that I really haven't started the Fast Diet yet because it has only been two days, and I am sure I lost a pound or two just for those two days. Unfortunately, while the logic is sound – you really will have lost a couple of pounds, so you can quit and still feel good about yourself – that is a trap you must stay clear of or you will never truly start.

After I weighed myself and found that I had not gained my weight back and I didn't look like I was walking around in a pup tent of lose skin I went back on the diet plan. I now weigh 205 pounds. I am quite happy at this weight, and I may or may not try to break the 200 pound barrier. If I do, it will not be for any cosmetic reasons, but just so I can put the big heavy block on 150, instead of starting with it on 200lbs.

I love to take naps. I always have. What I hate is waking up. The Fast Diet or any diet for that matter is the same way. The more often you quit the more times you have to start. Starting is hard. I know I am harping on this, I know I sound like a broken record, I know you are tired of it, but let me re-peat - starting is hard. Don't put yourself through that misery time after time, after all it is only for two weeks.

Once again, good luck to you. I know you hear this so of-ten that it is just a cliché' now, but if I can do it, you certainly can too.

Some Melon Nutritional Facts
Title: Watermelon
Serving Size 1 cup, balls (154g) 1 cup, diced (152g) 1 melon (15" long x 7 ½" diameter) (4518g) 1 wedge (approx 1/16 of melon) (286g) 10 watermelon balls (122g) 529g

Amount per serving

Calories 46 Calories from Fat 2

Total Fat 0g 0%

Saturated Fat 0g 0%

Cholesterol 0mg 0%

Sodium 2mg 0%

Total Carbohydrates 12g 4%

Dietary Fiber 1g

Sugars 10g

Protein 1g

Vitamin A 18%	Vitamin C 21%
Calcium 1%	Iron 2%
Thiamin 3%	Riboflavin 2%
Niacin 1%	Pantothenic Acid 3%
Vitamin B6 3%	Potassium 5%
Phosphorus 2%	Magnesium 4%
Zinc 1%	Copper 3%

* Percent Daily Values are based on a 2,000 calorie diet.
Show Daily Values Description:
46 calories, 1 gram of fiber, 1

Title: Cantaloupe

Serving Size   1 cup, balls (177g) 1 cup, cubes (160g) 1 cup, diced (156g) 1 melon, large (about 6 ½" diameter) (814g) 1 wedge, large (1/8 of large melon) (102g) 1 melon, medium (about 5" diameter) (552g) 1 wedge, medium (1/8 of medium melon) (69g) 1 melon, small (about 4-1/4" diameter) (441g) 1 wedge, small (1/8 of small melon) (55g) 10 cantaloupe balls (138g) 1 NLEA serving (134g)

Amount per serving

Calories 60 Calories from Fat 3

Total Fat 0g 0%

Saturated Fat 0g 0%

Cholesterol 0mg 0%

Sodium 28mg 1%

Total Carbohydrates 14g 5%

Dietary Fiber 2g

Sugars 14g

Protein 1g

Vitamin A 120% Vitamin C 108%

Calcium 2%   Iron 2%

Thiamin 5%   Riboflavin 2%

Niacin 6%   Pantothenic Acid 2%

Vitamin B6 6%   Potassium 14%

Phosphorus 3%   Magnesium 5%

Zinc 2%   Copper 4%

* Percent Daily Values are based on a 2,000 calorie diet.

60 calories in 1 cup of cantaloupe melon. An excellent source of vitamin A and vitamin C, a very good source of potassium, dietary fiber, vitamin B3 (niacin), vitamin B6 and folate. Contains such a high level of vitamin A that it can be used to prevent lung damage in smokers. It is an important weight loss and workout food.

Title: Honeydew Melon

Serving Size 1 cup, balls (177g) 1 cup, diced (approx 20 pieces per cup) (170g) 1 melon (5-1/4" diameter) (1000g) 1 melon (6" - 7" diameter) (1280g) 1 wedge (1/8 of 5-1/4" diameter melon) (125g) 1 wedge (1/8 of 6" to 7" diameter melon) (160g) 10 honeydew balls (138g) 1 NLEA serving (134g)

Amount per serving

Calories 64 Calories from Fat 2

Total Fat 0g 0%

Saturated Fat 0g 0%

Cholesterol 0mg 0%

Sodium 32mg 1%

Total Carbohydrates 16g 5%

Dietary Fiber 1g

Sugars 14g

Protein 1g

Vitamin A 2% Vitamin C 53%
Calcium 1% Iron 2%
Thiamin 4% Riboflavin 1%
Niacin 4% Pantothenic Acid 3%
Vitamin B6 8% Potassium 12%
Phosphorus 2% Magnesium 4%
Zinc 1% Copper 2%
* Percent Daily Values are based on a 2,000 calorie diet.

Chapter Four

Conclusions

Try and think of the Fast Diet as a weight loss work out plan.

Attempting this program during the summer will be much easier since during summer there is a much greater variety of melons from which to choose.

I did this in the winter for three reasons:

1. To prove a point that it can be accomplished at any time of the year. I must admit that there was a time or three, when I doubted the wisdom of this start date. I would have had a much easier time if I could have shaken things up with a casaba or Christmas melon. All I had to choose from were watermelon, cantaloupe, and honeydew. Many a time I had to eat under-ripe melons – my choices were limited. On the bright side it did keep me from over-eating.

2. This is when the mood hit me. If I waited until the summer I would not have started. As they say "Strike when the iron is *hot*".

3. I know I said that starting the Fast Diet would be easier in the summer. Unfortunately for me that is simply not true. The problem for me in starting during the summer is that I am first and foremost a Dad. I take off Tuesday and Thursday during the summers

to spend time with my kids while they are out of school. I have mentioned many times that it is easier to stick with the Fast Diet when I am at work. During the summer there are just too many temptations for me. For those of you who don't have the luxury of altering your schedule, I still think the summer is the easiest time since there is so much more variety to choose from.

After successfully having completed the Fast Diet myself, I began to approach patients and friends with my diet to have them try it and see what kind of results others could achieve. I have included some of their testimonials in the beginning of the book. More importantly though, is that a number of questions arose from the people who were considering starting, or were currently on my Fast Diet.

The most frequently asked question was how safe was the plan. I was actually a little startled by this question until I realized that almost everyone has been on some kind of diet before, however very few people have ever been on a Fast.

Again this plan is not truly a Fast. A true fast requires no caloric intake at all. If you are on a true fast you do need to be aware of overdoing it and depleting all of the energy and nutrition stored in your body. Since there is no true fasting with this plan the risk is no greater than any other diet out there.

The next most frequent question was how long will the weight stay off. This question is a bit trickier. The flip answer would be to just say that that is up to you. In all honesty it depends on many factors. Since everyone is different I can only use myself as an example. After the first time, I never did the Fast Diet in its pure form again. I did get on and off it again a few more times. However I did not do it hard core since I was already pretty much where I wanted to be. I did notice that after every time I stopped I would rebound about 3-4 pounds and then stay at that level. I mentioned earlier that I did add melon to my weekly diet to help me maintain my new weight and if I got on the scale and did not like what I saw I would just eat melon for one or two days and that tended to be all of the extra help I needed to maintain my new weight. The key was to weigh often so you could nip it in the bud.

Finally I was asked how often you can do it. This question actually made me happy to hear. It meant that a lot of people were so taken with this program for losing weight that they wanted to do it again and again. Happily the answer is as many times as you like. If you are following the plan and taking the breaks and eating on the days that you are supposed to there is no limit as to the number of times you can start the Fast Diet.

If you had any doubts I hope that this clarifies them. I am well aware that anything new needs to prove itself. That is why whenever possible I have used myself as an example and tried to answer any foreseeable questions that might arise.

Testimonials:

I am 26 years old and the current Middle weight champion in Mixed Martial Arts. Losing weight fast without losing strength is essential in my profession. Typically I need to cut 35 lbs before my fights. When Dr. Smith asked me to try his "Fast Diet" for two weeks, I was skeptical but willing. Now I use his plan before all of my fights and recommend it to anyone who needs to lose weight fast,

Danny "Badboy" Babcock

As a woman rapidly approaching middle age I have found it harder and harder to lose weight. I decided to give Dr. Smith's "Fast Diet" a try and lost 7lbs in the first 3 days! At the end of the two week period, I was very pleased with the results. Since then I have highly recommended this diet to many of my friends.

Jennifer Corvino

I have struggled with weight issues most of my life. I've tried different weight loss products and workout programs including joining a gym, all with not much success. But when Dr. Smith told me about his "Fast Diet" and that exercise was not required, I was curious. After Dr. Smith explained what the "Fast diet" was, I decided to try it for the full two week period. For my two cheat days, I continued eating the watermelon for breakfast and lunch, but added fish and vegetables for dinner. I am now happy to tell you that I have lost a total of eleven pounds and am continuing on to the next ten. For all of those who decide to try this, I wish you much success.

Deb G.

Port St. Lucie, Florida

www.ingramcontent.com/pod-product-compliance
Lightning Source LLC
Chambersburg PA
CBHW060641290526
45793CB00001B/342